RICE DIET FOR BEGINNERS GUIDE

The Complete Guide to Using and Maximizing Rice Diet to Shed Excess Weight and Nourish your Body Including Rice Diet Meal Plan

Mina Mong
Copyright@2024

TABLE OF CONTENT

CHAPTER 1

INTRODUCTION

In a world filled with ever-changing diet trends, the rice diet has proven itself as a reliable method for achieving weight loss and improving overall health. The rice diet has gained attention for its simplicity, effectiveness, and potential health benefits, stemming from the work of Dr. Walter Kempner in the mid-20th century. This introduction offers a thorough exploration of the rice diet, including its historical background, the principles it follows, and its goal of promoting both weight loss and nourishment.

1.1 Introduction to the Rice Diet

The origins of the rice diet can be traced back to the Duke University Medical Center in the 1930s. Dr. Walter Kempner, a physician and researcher, developed this diet as a therapeutic approach for individuals with hypertension and kidney disease. Over time, its uses have gone beyond just medical conditions and now encompass weight management and overall well-being.

The diet developed by Dr. Kempner, called the Rice Diet Program, focused heavily on incorporating rice as a main component, along with an abundance of fruits and vegetables. The deliberate simplicity of this approach was designed to limit the intake of sodium, fat, and protein, with the aim of lowering blood pressure and encouraging weight loss.

1.2 Purpose and Benefits

The main objective of the rice diet is twofold: achieving weight loss and providing nourishment. Although weight loss is a common objective for many people, the rice diet also prioritizes the provision of vital nutrients to promote overall well-being. Contrary to trendy diets that prioritize quick weight loss, the rice diet promotes a comprehensive approach that values a well-rounded and enduring lifestyle.

One of the main advantages of the rice diet is its ability to act as a rejuvenating cleanse for the body. Opting for whole grains such as brown rice instead of refined alternatives allows individuals to unlock the nutritional goodness of these foods, reaping the rewards of fiber, vitamins, and minerals. In addition, the diet's emphasis on low-calorie, low-fat, and low-sodium foods is in line with heart-healthy principles and could potentially enhance metabolic function.

1.3 Important Notice and Health Considerations

Prior to making any substantial adjustments to your diet, it is important to recognize that everyone's health requirements differ. It's important to exercise caution when considering the rice diet, as it may not be suitable for everyone. This is particularly true for individuals with underlying health conditions or specific nutritional needs.

Please note that this guide should not be considered a replacement for advice from a qualified medical professional. Prior to embarking on the rice diet or any other weight loss program, it is highly advisable to seek guidance from a healthcare professional or a registered dietitian. They offer personalized guidance tailored to an individual's health history, current medical conditions, and nutritional needs.

In the sections that follow, we will explore the principles of the rice diet in greater detail. We will discuss the types of rice that are recommended, the significance of maintaining a balanced intake of macronutrients, the incorporation of nutrient-rich foods, and practical strategies for effectively managing weight and promoting overall nourishment. Embarking on a path towards a more wholesome way of living starts with grasping the fundamentals of the rice diet and customizing its principles to suit personal needs and preferences.

CHAPTER 2

Understanding the Rice Diet

Exploring the path to a more wholesome way of living often requires understanding the nuances of different dietary approaches. The rice diet, with its origins in the mid-20th century and influenced by the groundbreaking research of Dr. Walter Kempner, has become a unique method for achieving weight loss and improving overall health. Here, we explore the fundamental principles that shape the rice diet, exploring its historical background, the scientific reasoning behind its creation, and the various ways it affects the body.

2.1 Understanding the Fundamentals of the Rice Diet Philosophy

The rice diet philosophy is centered around the concept of simplicity and restriction. Contrary to popular diets that require complicated meal plans or cutting out entire food groups, the rice diet focuses on a select few essential elements. It is recommended to incorporate rice, particularly brown rice due to its superior nutritional content, into your diet. Additionally, make sure to include a variety of fruits and vegetables as part of your regular meals. These foods are the cornerstone of a healthy diet, offering vital nutrients while keeping calories, sodium, and fat in check.

The rice diet is intentionally designed to be simple. It provides a refreshing break from the frequently overwhelming and complex realm of contemporary diets, presenting a simple and straightforward approach that aligns with the traditional diets of various cultures. By focusing on a diet that prioritizes easily digestible and nutrient-dense foods such as rice, individuals strive to attain weight loss and enhance their overall health without the hassle of complex meal planning or calorie counting.

2.2 Different Varieties of Rice and Their Nutritional Values

When it comes to rice, there are significant differences in quality and taste. Having a deep understanding of the nutritional variations among different types of rice is essential for optimizing the advantages of the rice diet. When it comes to rice, brown rice is a standout choice. It has intact bran and germ layers, which means it's packed with fiber, essential vitamins, and minerals. It's important to note that this food option offers a steady supply of energy and helps promote a sense of fullness, which can be beneficial for individuals aiming to lose weight.

White rice, however, goes through a processing method that eliminates the bran and germ, resulting in a loss of certain nutrients. White rice, although a source of energy, does not contain the same amount of fiber and micronutrients as brown rice.

Emphasizing the importance of incorporating whole grains into your diet, the rice diet aims to maximize the nutritional advantages for both weight management and overall well-being.

2.3 Exploring the Benefits of the Rice Diet for Weight Loss

The weight loss aspect of the rice diet is a result of various factors, including the combination of controlled calorie consumption, lower sodium content, and the natural properties of whole grains. By emphasizing foods that are low in fat and calories, individuals who are knowledgeable about nutrition understand the importance of creating a calorie deficit, which is a key principle in achieving weight loss.

Adding brown rice and other whole grains can boost the effectiveness of the diet for weight loss. Whole grains are packed with dietary fiber, which not only supports a healthy digestive system but also helps you feel satisfied. Understanding the satiety factor is crucial for managing portion sizes and cutting down on calories.

In addition, the rice diet's limitation on sodium has been associated with decreased water retention and bloating, resulting in an initial increase in weight loss that surpasses the loss of body fat. The combination of these factors creates a comprehensive approach to weight management, with the diet focusing on both the quantity and quality of food consumed.

In addition to its potential weight loss effects, the rice diet may offer various other health benefits. According to some experts, following this diet may potentially enhance insulin sensitivity and promote cardiovascular well-being. It is worth mentioning that people may have different reactions to the diet, and further research is required to gain a comprehensive understanding of its impact on long-term health.

In the following sections of this guide, we will delve into the practical aspects of embracing the rice diet. This will include tips on selecting the perfect rice, ensuring a well-rounded intake of macronutrients, incorporating nourishing foods, and creating sustainable meal plans. With a deep knowledge of the principles behind the rice diet, individuals can make well-informed choices to achieve their weight loss and nourishment goals.

CHAPTER 3

Choosing the Right Rice

Choosing the right type of rice is crucial for achieving weight loss and maintaining good health as part of the rice diet. Here, we explore the intricacies of choosing the perfect rice, examining the nutritional variations among different types and uncovering the effects these choices have on the body.

When it comes to the battle between brown rice and white rice, there are a few key differences to consider. Brown rice, with its nutty flavor and chewy texture, is a whole grain that retains its bran and germ layers. This means it's packed with fiber, vitamins, and minerals. On the other hand, white rice has had its bran and germ layers removed, resulting in a milder taste and softer texture. While white rice may be

The discussion surrounding brown rice versus white rice is at the heart of the rice diet philosophy. Although both types come from the same grain, they undergo varying degrees of processing, which leads to different nutritional profiles.

The Nutrient-Rich Powerhouse: Brown Rice

Many people consider brown rice to be a more nutritionally dense option because it retains its outer layers—the bran and germ—during the milling process. The preservation of the whole grain offers notable nutritional benefits. Brown rice is a fantastic choice for those looking to improve their digestive health, feel satisfied after meals, and maintain stable blood sugar levels. Brown rice is a great option for people who are watching their weight or have concerns about insulin sensitivity, thanks to its high fiber content. This can help slow down the release of glucose in the body.

Brown rice is not only rich in fiber, but it also boasts a variety of essential nutrients like magnesium, phosphorus, and B vitamins, including B6 and niacin. These essential nutrients play a crucial role in supporting different aspects of our body, such as maintaining energy levels, promoting strong bones, and supporting overall neurological health. The inclusion of antioxidants in the bran layer enhances the health advantages, as they effectively counteract oxidative stress and inflammation.

White Rice: A Staple with Considerations

On the other hand, white rice goes through a milling process where the bran and germ layers are removed, resulting in only the endosperm remaining. Through this processing method, certain nutrients are removed from the whole grain, leading to a final product that contains less fiber, vitamins, and minerals when compared to its brown counterpart.

White rice may be a convenient and fast source of energy, but it falls short in terms of nutritional value compared to brown rice. White rice is known for its ability to quickly break down and be absorbed by the body, which can cause blood sugar levels to rise rapidly. This may have an effect on how sensitive the body is to insulin. White rice may not be the best option for those looking to manage their weight or individuals with diabetes-related concerns.

It is important to keep in mind that the rice diet does not completely eliminate white rice, but rather promotes a thoughtful and well-rounded approach. For those who are not dealing with any specific health issues, it may be alright to include white rice in their diet in moderation. It's crucial to have a deep understanding of the nutritional trade-offs and make well-informed choices that align with your personal health goals.

3.2 Other Whole Grain Options

As a connoisseur of cuisine, it's always exciting to venture beyond the realm of brown rice and discover a plethora of whole grain alternatives. Not only does this bring a delightful variety to your meals, but it also elevates your nutritional intake to new heights. Incorporating whole grains like quinoa, wild rice, barley, and bulgur into your diet can be a great way to enhance your meals. Every single one of these grains offers a distinct array of nutrients, making them valuable additions to a balanced and varied diet.

3.2.1 Quinoa: The Ultimate Protein Source

Quinoa is truly remarkable, as it is not only a whole grain but also a complete protein, containing all the essential amino acids. Quinoa is a fantastic option for those who follow vegetarian or vegan diets, as it offers a protein source that rivals animal products.

Furthermore, quinoa boasts an impressive nutritional profile, packed with fiber, iron, magnesium, and antioxidants. This makes it an excellent choice to enhance the nutritional value of any rice-based meal.

3.2.2 Wild Rice: A Delectable and Nutrient-Packed Option

Wild rice is a whole grain that boasts a unique texture and a delightful nutty flavor. It also provides a range of nutritional benefits. This particular food item provides a significant amount of fiber, as well as important minerals like phosphorus and magnesium. Additionally, it contains antioxidants that are beneficial for overall health. Wild rice offers a distinct flavor that can bring a delightful twist to your meals, elevating your culinary journey and promoting your health objectives.

3.2.3 Barley: A Nutritious Choice for a Healthy Heart

Barley is a fantastic whole grain that offers remarkable advantages for maintaining a healthy heart. This particular ingredient is rich in beta-glucans, a type of soluble fiber known for its cholesterol-lowering properties. Barley is a fantastic source of essential vitamins and minerals, such as niacin, selenium, and phosphorus. Barley is known for its high fiber content, which can help you feel fuller for longer and support a healthy digestive system.

Bulgur: A Versatile Grain That Cooks Quickly

Bulgur is a popular ingredient in Middle Eastern cuisine. It is a type of cracked wheat that has undergone parboiling and drying. This whole grain cooks quickly and has a mild flavor, making it a convenient choice for a variety of dishes. Bulgur is packed with fiber, manganese, and magnesium, which contribute to a healthy digestive system and overall wellness.

Adding a range of whole grains to your rice diet can boost nutritional diversity and make your meals more enjoyable and fulfilling. Exploring various grains enables people to uncover their personal preferences while enjoying the wide range of health advantages provided by whole grains.

3.3 Guidelines for Portion Control

Proper selection of rice and other whole grains is important, but it's essential to remember the importance of portion control when following the rice diet. When it comes to achieving weight loss goals, it's crucial to keep track of the calories you consume and have a good grasp of portion sizes. This way, you can find the right balance between nourishing your body and practicing moderation.

A typical serving of cooked rice is usually around 1/2 to 1 cup. This serving size offers a balanced amount of carbohydrates, as well as fiber and vital nutrients. Keep in mind that portion sizes may differ depending on various factors like age, activity level, and metabolic rate. Customizing portion sizes to meet individual needs and goals promotes a personalized and long-lasting approach to the rice diet.

Ultimately, the selection of rice in the rice diet goes beyond personal preference. It is a calculated choice that plays a crucial role in establishing the nutritional basis of the entire dietary plan. Choosing nutrient-rich alternatives such as brown rice and incorporating a range of whole grains can help individuals achieve weight loss, enhance overall health, and embark on a path towards optimal well-being. In the upcoming sections of this guide, we will delve into the significance of maintaining a well-balanced diet, incorporating foods that are packed with essential nutrients, and implementing effective strategies for managing weight successfully while following the rice diet.

CHAPTER 4

Balanced Macronutrients in the Rice Diet

When it comes to achieving sustainable weight loss and overall well-being, the rice diet places a strong focus on attaining a harmonious balance of macronutrients. Understanding the importance of macronutrients is essential for maintaining a balanced and nourishing diet. Here, we explore the significance of every macronutrient, their functions in the body, and the way a well-rounded approach contributes to the effectiveness of the rice diet.

4.1 The Significance of a Well-Balanced Macronutrient Profile

Macronutrients play a crucial role in our diet as they provide the energy needed for important physiological functions. It is essential to maintain a proper balance of proteins, carbohydrates, and fats in order to support bodily functions, promote satiety, and ensure overall health. Understanding the importance of macronutrient balance is key to maximizing nutrition and achieving weight loss goals.

4.1.1 Proteins: Essential for a Healthy Body

Proteins play a crucial role in the body, supporting tissue repair and maintenance, enzyme and hormone synthesis, and immune system function. When it comes to the rice diet, it's crucial to include lean sources of protein. Not only does it help maintain muscle mass, but it also supports the body's metabolic functions and keeps you feeling satisfied.

There are various sources of protein that can be incorporated into a rice-based diet, such as poultry, fish, tofu, legumes, and beans. These choices not only fulfill the body's protein requirements, but also provide an array of essential nutrients like iron, zinc, and various vitamins. By selecting lean protein sources, individuals can adhere to a calorie-conscious approach while still fulfilling their protein needs.

4.1.2 Carbohydrates: The Body's Main Source of Energy

Carbohydrates play a crucial role in fueling the body, providing the necessary energy for daily activities and exercise. When it comes to the rice diet, whole grains like brown rice are the star of the show, providing a reliable source of complex carbohydrates. When it comes to carbohydrates, whole grains are the way to go. Unlike those sugary simple carbs, complex carbohydrates found in whole grains are digested at a slower pace, resulting in a steady release of glucose and a long-lasting energy boost.

Although the rice diet focuses on reducing calorie consumption, it does not promote the complete removal of carbohydrates. Instead, it promotes the consumption of nutrient-rich,

high-fiber carbohydrates that help you feel
satisfied, promote a healthy digestive system,
and provide important vitamins and minerals.

The Importance of Fats in Maintaining Health
and Absorbing Nutrients

Understanding the importance of fats in our
diet is crucial. They play a vital role in helping
our bodies absorb fat-soluble vitamins like A, D,
E, and K. Additionally, fats are necessary for
maintaining cell structure and regulating
important bodily processes. When it comes to
the rice diet, the main emphasis is on including
nutritious fats while keeping a check on
saturated and trans fats. There are a variety of
options when it comes to incorporating healthy
fats into your diet. Some examples include
avocados, nuts, seeds, and olive oil.

Adding fats to your diet can help you feel more
satisfied and prevent you from snacking too
much or overeating. Understanding the

nutritional value of different food components is crucial for maintaining a well-rounded diet. Although fats contain more calories compared to proteins and carbohydrates, their role in nutrient absorption and overall well-being cannot be overlooked.

4.2 Protein Content in the Rice Diet

Proteins play a crucial role in the rice diet for various reasons. They help in preserving muscle, boosting metabolism, and keeping you feeling satisfied. By selecting lean sources of protein, individuals can fulfill their nutritional requirements while adhering to the calorie-conscious approach of the rice diet.

4.2.1 Poultry and Fish: Optimal Protein Choices

Lean sources of protein, like poultry and fish, are a perfect fit for the rice diet. These choices offer a great source of protein without an excessive amount of saturated fat. Fish, especially, provides extra advantages due to its omega-3 fatty acids, which are renowned for their positive effects on heart health and reducing inflammation.

Integrating poultry and fish into your meals brings a delightful burst of flavors and a touch of diversity, transforming the rice diet into a sustainable and pleasurable dietary choice. Opting for grilled, baked, or steamed preparations is recommended over cooking methods that involve excessive frying or added fats.

Exploring Plant-Based Protein Alternatives

If you're looking to follow a plant-based or vegetarian version of the rice diet, incorporating tofu, legumes, and beans into your meals can provide you with a great source of protein. Tofu is a highly versatile ingredient that has the amazing ability to soak up flavors, making it perfect for all sorts of culinary masterpieces.

Legumes and beans, such as lentils, chickpeas, and black beans, offer a wealth of protein along with a generous dose of dietary fiber, vitamins, and minerals. This combination provides excellent support for digestive health, helps you feel satisfied after meals, and boosts the nutritional value of your dishes.

4.3 Embracing Nutritious Carbohydrates

Choosing high-quality, whole grains is essential for maximizing the nutritional benefits of the rice diet, as carbohydrates play a crucial role in this eating plan. These carbohydrates offer long-lasting energy, support digestive health, and contribute to overall well-being.

4.3.1 Whole Grains: The Cornerstone of the Rice Diet

The rice diet's carbohydrate content is built upon a foundation of whole grains, including brown rice, quinoa, wild rice, and barley. The fiber, vitamins, and minerals found in these grains are preserved due to the intact bran and germ layers, unlike in refined grains where they are often lost during processing.

Brown rice is a fantastic choice for those looking to feel satisfied and promote a healthy digestive system. Adding quinoa to your meals not only enhances their nutritional value, but also brings a delightful depth of flavor. Meanwhile, incorporating wild rice and barley not only adds a unique taste to your dishes, but also provides additional health benefits.

The Incredible Nutritional Value of Fruits and Vegetables

Alongside whole grains, fruits and vegetables are essential components rich in carbohydrates that are vital for the rice diet. These foods are packed with all the necessary vitamins, minerals, antioxidants, and dietary fiber your body needs.

Indulge in the delightful flavors and numerous health advantages of fruits like berries, apples, and citrus fruits. Including a variety of vegetables in your meals can greatly enhance their nutritional value.

It is highly recommended to incorporate a wide range of fruits and vegetables into the rice diet in order to maximize the intake of essential nutrients. These plant-based carbohydrates add a delightful variety of flavors, textures, and colors to meals, enhancing their overall appeal.

4.4 Incorporating Vital Fats

When it comes to the rice diet, the main emphasis is on including nutritious fats that promote overall health and well-being.

Understanding the importance of essential fats is crucial for a well-rounded understanding of nutrition. These fats are not only involved in nutrient absorption, but also play a vital role in hormone production and cellular function.

They are not only packed with nutrients, but also have a wonderfully creamy texture that adds a touch of indulgence to any dish.

Avocados are renowned for their velvety texture and indulgent taste, making them a top choice for those seeking a nourishing source of monounsaturated fats. These fats have been linked to promoting heart health and can help you feel fuller for longer. Avocados are packed with vital nutrients like potassium, vitamin K, and folate.

Incorporating sliced avocados into salads, spreading them on whole-grain toast, or using them in various dishes can greatly enhance the nutritional value and overall enjoyment of the rice diet.

4.4.2 Nuts and Seeds: A Delicious and Nutritious Option

These nutrient-rich powerhouses, such as almonds, walnuts, chia seeds, and flaxseeds, offer a wealth of healthy fats, protein, and a variety of essential vitamins and minerals. These delectable options can be effortlessly incorporated into your yogurt, salads, or enjoyed as delightful snacks.

When adding nuts and seeds to your rice diet, it's important to consider portion sizes.

It is crucial to exercise control when it comes to their calorie density. Indulging in a modest portion offers a delightful crispness and a plethora of healthful advantages.

Olive Oil: A Versatile Cooking Companion

Olive oil, particularly extra virgin olive oil, is a fundamental component of the Mediterranean diet and perfectly complements the principles of the rice diet. This particular food is abundant in monounsaturated fats and is packed with antioxidants that possess anti-inflammatory properties.

Utilizing olive oil in your culinary endeavors can elevate the taste of your dishes, all the while offering a nourishing dose of beneficial fats. Its incredible versatility makes it an invaluable addition to any kitchen, especially for those who are following a rice-based diet.

4.5 Achieving a Harmonious Approach to Sustainable Nutrition

Finding the perfect balance of macronutrients goes beyond just choosing the right foods. It also involves carefully considering portion sizes and overall energy intake. With a focus on whole grains, lean proteins, and healthy fats, the rice diet offers a great way for individuals to craft well-rounded and enjoyable meals.

Having a well-balanced mix of macronutrients is crucial for maintaining steady energy levels, promoting healthy metabolism, and avoiding drastic spikes and drops in blood sugar. Adopting this well-rounded approach also helps in reaching and sustaining a healthy weight by encouraging a sense of satisfaction and avoiding excessive eating.

In addition, maintaining a well-balanced diet is crucial for obtaining a diverse range of vital nutrients, which in turn supports overall well-being and helps prevent nutritional deficiencies. The delicate balance of macronutrients in the rice diet results in a harmonious combination that amplifies the advantages of weight loss and nourishment.

In the following sections of this guide, we will delve into the practical aspects of meal planning within the rice diet framework. This will include providing sample meal plans, offering cooking tips, and suggesting innovative ways to incorporate nutrient-rich foods. With a deep understanding of the principles of balanced macronutrients, individuals can embark on their rice diet journey with a sense of knowledge, purpose, and a focus on long-term well-being.

CHAPTER 5

Exploring Nutrient-Rich Foods

When it comes to leading a healthier lifestyle and maintaining overall well-being, it's crucial to focus on incorporating foods that are packed with essential nutrients. Consuming foods that are packed with essential vitamins and minerals can provide the body with the necessary fuel to maintain vitality, support a strong immune system, and effectively manage weight. Within this section, we will explore the concept of nutrient-rich foods, delving into different categories, their advantages, and practical methods for integrating them into your diet.

5.1 Vegetables: A Multitude of Nutritional Benefits

Vegetables truly shine as essential components of a well-balanced and nourishing diet, providing a plethora of vital nutrients, including vitamins, minerals, fiber, and antioxidants. Exploring a wide array of vegetables allows for a rich assortment of nutrients that support overall well-being.

Dark leafy greens are incredibly nutritious and packed with essential vitamins and minerals. They are true powerhouses when it comes to providing our bodies with the nutrients they need to thrive.

Dark leafy greens like spinach, kale, Swiss chard, and collard greens are incredibly nutritious. These greens are rich in vitamins A, C, and K, along with minerals such as iron and calcium, which help boost immune function, promote bone health, and contribute to overall well-being.

Adding dark leafy greens to your salads, stir-fries, or smoothies can bring a burst of color and a healthy dose of nutrients to your meals.

These greens are not only great for digestion, but they also help you feel satisfied.

Cruciferous Vegetables: Powerful Allies Packed with Antioxidants

These vegetables, like broccoli, cauliflower, Brussels sprouts, and cabbage, are renowned for their impressive antioxidant properties. These vegetables are packed with compounds that can help your body with detoxification and potentially even have anti-cancer properties.

Preparing cruciferous vegetables through steaming, roasting, or sautéing can bring out their delicious flavors without compromising their nutritional value. Ensuring a wide range of colors and textures in your vegetable choices is key to maximizing the nutritional benefits.

Colorful Bell Peppers: A Healthy Dose of Vitamin C

Bell peppers, in their vibrant array of colors, are packed with vitamin C. This powerful antioxidant not only boosts the immune system, but also promotes healthy skin and aids in the absorption of iron from plant-based sources. Bell peppers are a fantastic source of fiber and a variety of essential vitamins, including vitamin A and B-complex vitamins.

Adding bell peppers to salads, fajitas, or stir-fries enhances the taste and nutritional value. Their inherent sweetness perfectly complements a variety of dishes.

5.2 Fruits: A Delectable Source of Essential Nutrients

Fruits provide a wonderful balance of sweetness and nourishment, offering a wide range of vitamins, minerals, fiber, and antioxidants. Incorporating a diverse range of fruits into your diet not only satisfies your cravings for something sweet, but also promotes optimal health.

5.2.1 Berries: Nutritional Powerhouses

It's widely known that berries, like blueberries, strawberries, raspberries, and blackberries, are highly regarded for their impressive antioxidant levels. Antioxidants play a crucial role in fighting oxidative stress and inflammation, which are important for maintaining cellular health and promoting longevity.

Berries are incredibly versatile when it comes to enhancing your meals. Whether you enjoy them in yogurt, smoothies, or as a delicious topping for oatmeal, these little gems add a burst of flavor and a healthy dose of nutrition to your diet. Their inherent sweetness eliminates the necessity for additional sugars.

Citrus fruits are packed with essential nutrients like vitamin C and fiber.

Did you know that citrus fruits like oranges, grapefruits, lemons, and limes are packed with vitamin C? This essential nutrient is known for its ability to boost immune function and promote collagen synthesis. Citrus fruits are known for their beneficial effects on digestion and blood sugar levels.

Indulging in citrus fruits as snacks or adding them to salads and desserts offers a delightful explosion of flavor while also providing a nourishing boost of nutrients. With the wide range of citrus fruits available, there are endless possibilities for culinary experimentation.

5.2.3 Apples and Pears: Fiber-Rich Choices

Apples and pears are fantastic choices for maintaining a healthy digestive system and feeling satisfied after a meal. These fruits are packed with essential vitamins, minerals, and antioxidants that promote overall health and vitality.

Adding sliced apples with nut butter or pear slices to salads can provide a delightful combination of crunch and sweetness, all while keeping the calorie count in check. It is worth noting that incorporating the skin of these fruits can significantly boost their fiber content.

5.3 Dairy or Alternatives: Enhancing Bone Health and More

Consuming dairy products and dairy alternatives is crucial for obtaining vital nutrients like calcium, vitamin D, and protein. These nutrients play a vital role in maintaining strong bones, supporting muscle function, and ensuring a healthy metabolic balance.

5.3.1 Healthy Dairy Choices: Boosting Calcium and Protein Intake

Opt for low-fat or non-fat dairy options like milk, yogurt, and cheese, which provide a good amount of calcium and protein. Understanding the importance of calcium for bone health and protein for muscle maintenance and repair is crucial.

Adding dairy to your diet can be effortless, like savoring a cup of yogurt with fresh fruit or sprinkling some cheese onto a salad. Opting for low-fat or non-fat options is in line with the calorie-conscious approach of the rice diet.

Exploring Dairy Alternatives: Embracing the Power of Plants
For those with dietary restrictions or preferences, there are a variety of dairy alternatives available that provide a wealth of nutrients. Options like almond milk, soy milk, and coconut milk can be excellent substitutes. Several of these alternatives are enriched with calcium and vitamin D to replicate the nutritional composition of dairy products.

Incorporating non-dairy options into your smoothies, cereal, or coffee can add a velvety consistency and enhance your overall nutritional intake. It is important to carefully read labels to ensure that all the necessary nutrients are included in the food.

5.4 Protein Sources: Building and Repairing Tissues

Protein plays a vital role in the rice diet, helping to maintain muscle, support the immune system, and promote a sense of satiety. It is important to incorporate a diverse range of protein sources into your diet to ensure a balanced and nourishing intake of nutrients.

5.4.1 Lean Poultry: High-Quality Protein

Poultry, like chicken and turkey, is a popular choice for protein in the rice diet. These choices offer a great source of protein that is low in saturated fat, which is important for maintaining muscle and supporting overall metabolic function.

For a well-rounded meal, consider combining grilled, baked, or roasted poultry dishes with whole grains and vegetables. Adding herbs and spices to your dishes can enhance the taste without adding unnecessary calories.

5.4.2 Fish: Promoting Heart Health with Omega-3 Fatty Acids

Fish is a fantastic choice for those looking to improve their heart health and reduce inflammation. Not only is it a great source of protein, but it is also rich in omega-3 fatty acids, which have numerous benefits for the body. Salmon, mackerel, and trout are excellent sources of omega-3s, which are highly beneficial for your health.

Adding fish to your meals, whether grilled, baked, or broiled, brings a delightful range of flavors and boosts the nutritional value of your diet. Incorporating fish into your diet at least twice a week is in line with dietary guidelines for promoting heart health.

Plant-Based Proteins: Tofu, Legumes, and Beans

If you're looking to incorporate more plant-based protein into your diet, there are plenty of nutrient-rich alternatives to choose from. Tofu, legumes, and beans are all excellent options. Did you know that tofu, which is derived from soybeans, is a fantastic source of complete protein? On the other hand, legumes and beans offer a wealth of fiber, vitamins, and minerals.

Bean salads, lentil soups, or tofu stir-fries are excellent examples of how plant-based proteins can be incredibly versatile. By incorporating these choices alongside whole grains, you can achieve a well-rounded amino acid profile.

5.5 Whole Grains: Nourishing Sources of Energy and Fiber

Whole grains like brown rice, quinoa, and oats form the basis of the rice diet. These carbohydrate sources are packed with nutrients, offering long-lasting energy and a wide range of essential vitamins and minerals.

Brown Rice: A Nutritional Powerhouse

Brown rice is a highly nutritious whole grain, thanks to its intact bran and germ layers. This food is rich in fiber, B vitamins, and important minerals like magnesium and phosphorus. The high fiber content in this food not only promotes healthy digestion, but also helps you feel satisfied and full.

Adding brown rice to your meals, whether as a side dish or a foundation for stir-fries and grain bowls, elevates the nutritional value of your diet. Exploring various whole grains can bring a delightful range of flavors and textures to your meals.

The Versatility and Nutritional Benefits of Quinoa

Quinoa is a highly versatile whole grain that is known for being a complete protein source. This particular option is a great source of plant-based protein, as it contains all the essential amino acids. Quinoa boasts an impressive nutritional profile, packed with fiber, iron, and magnesium.

Incorporating quinoa into salads, as a side dish, or as a foundation for grain bowls brings a wealth of nutrients and a delightful texture. With its quick cooking time, it's the perfect option for those with busy schedules.

A delicious and nutritious breakfast choice: oats, a heart-healthy option.

Oats are an excellent choice for those looking to improve their heart health. This wholesome grain is packed with beta-glucans, a type of soluble fiber that has been proven to lower cholesterol levels. Oats are a fantastic source of B vitamins, iron, and antioxidants.

Beginning your day with a nourishing breakfast option like oatmeal or adding oats to smoothies and baked goods can provide a wholesome and nutritious start. There are different types of oats that can be used in various culinary applications, offering flexibility and versatility.

5.6 Nuts and Seeds: Nutrient-Rich Snacking

Including almonds, walnuts, chia seeds, and flaxseeds in your diet can provide you with a wealth of nutrients. These options are packed with healthy fats, protein, and a variety of essential vitamins and minerals. Although they are high in calories, they provide various health benefits when eaten in moderation.

5.6.1 Almonds: A Healthy Choice for Snacking

Almonds are packed with nutrients like monounsaturated fats, vitamin E, and magnesium, which contribute to their status as a heart-healthy snack choice. Almonds are known for their ability to keep you feeling full and satisfied, thanks to their healthy fats and protein content.

Adding a small handful of almonds to your snack or incorporating them into yogurt and salads can give you a delightful crunch while also providing you with nutritional benefits. Choosing unsalted almonds is a great way to make a heart-healthy decision.

Chia Seeds: A Nutritional Powerhouse

Chia seeds are incredibly nutritious, offering a wealth of omega-3 fatty acids, fiber, and a variety of essential vitamins and minerals. Their ability to transform into a gel-like consistency when immersed in liquid makes them incredibly versatile for enhancing a wide range of dishes.

Incorporating chia seeds into your smoothies, yogurt, or overnight oats can elevate the nutritional value and improve the overall texture of your meals. Their capacity to soak up liquid enhances the sensation of satiety.

5.7 Hydration: The Key to Efficient Nutrient Transport

Proper hydration is an essential part of maintaining a well-balanced diet. Proper hydration is crucial for the optimal functioning of our bodies, as it facilitates the transportation of vital nutrients and aids in digestion. Ensuring proper hydration is crucial for maintaining optimal energy levels, cognitive function, and skin health.

Water: The Best Way to Stay Hydrated

Water is the ultimate and most essential source of hydration. It's absolutely crucial for your body to function properly, helping with nutrient absorption, temperature regulation, and waste elimination.

Adding water-rich foods like fruits and vegetables can enhance hydration levels. Staying hydrated is crucial for maintaining optimal health, and one way to achieve this is by sipping water consistently throughout the day, even between meals.

5.8 Crafting Well-Balanced and Nourishing Meals

Mastering the art of creating a well-rounded and nourishing diet requires careful consideration when selecting meals and incorporating a diverse range of food options. Here are some practical strategies for crafting meals that are both satisfying and nourishing within the context of the rice diet:

5.8.1 Emphasize the Importance of Whole Grains in Your Meals

Emphasizing the use of whole grains like brown rice, quinoa, or oats in your meals provides a solid base packed with complex carbohydrates, fiber, and vital nutrients. These grains are excellent for providing long-lasting energy and promoting a satisfying feeling of fullness.

Focus on incorporating lean proteins into your diet.

Including lean protein sources like poultry, fish, tofu, legumes, or beans in your diet can help maintain muscle, support metabolic function, and provide a balanced amino acid profile.

Incorporating both plant-based and animal-based proteins into your meals can bring a delightful range of flavors and textures.

5.8.3 Emphasize the Importance of Vegetables

It is important to include a generous amount of vegetables in every meal. Their nutritional value, including fiber, vitamins, minerals, and antioxidants, not only promotes good health but also enhances the presentation of a well-balanced meal. Exploring different cooking techniques and seasonings can greatly enhance the taste of vegetables.

5.8.4 Emphasize the Addition of Fruits for a Naturally Sweet Flavor

Incorporating a diverse range of fruits into your meals or savoring them as snacks offers a delightful burst of natural sweetness, while also delivering a wealth of essential vitamins, minerals, and antioxidants. There are so many delicious ways to enjoy fruits - you can add them to salads, create delightful yogurt parfaits, or simply savor them on their own for a refreshing and tasty treat.

Embrace the inclusion of healthy fats in your diet.

Adding sources of healthy fats like avocados, nuts, seeds, and olive oil can enhance the flavor, provide a feeling of fullness, and supply essential nutrients to your meals. It is important to be mindful of portion sizes because fats have a higher calorie density. However, incorporating fats into your diet can contribute to a balanced and nutritious eating plan.

Practice Mindful Eating

Practicing mindful eating entails fully immersing yourself in the dining experience, relishing every morsel, and tuning in to your body's signals of hunger and satisfaction. Embracing this approach encourages a positive connection with food, discourages excessive consumption, and supports overall health and happiness.

5.9 Moderation and Variety: Essential for a Balanced Diet

Understanding the importance of a balanced diet, it is crucial to incorporate a wide range of nutritious foods while also practicing portion control. It is important to note that no single food can fully meet all of our nutritional needs. To ensure that we receive a wide range of essential nutrients, it is recommended to maintain a diverse and varied diet that includes a variety of vitamins, minerals, and antioxidants.

It's important to keep in mind portion sizes and find a balance between the calories you consume and the energy you burn. One can savor a diverse array of delectable dishes without imposing unnecessary limitations.

CHAPTER 6

Nourishing the Body with Vital Fluids

One must carefully manage their fluid intake and output to ensure the body has enough water for vital physiological processes. In this comprehensive examination of hydration, we will explore the vital role that water plays in supporting the human body, identify common indicators of dehydration, analyze the various factors that can impact an individual's hydration requirements, and provide practical tips for effectively managing fluid levels to ensure optimal balance.

1. The Importance of Staying Hydrated

Water is an essential element of the human body, making up a substantial portion of body weight. Understanding the importance of various physiological processes is crucial as they play a vital role in nutrient transport, temperature regulation, digestion, and waste elimination. Proper hydration is absolutely essential for maintaining the delicate balance of bodily fluids, supporting optimal cellular function, and ensuring the smooth operation of all our organs and systems.

2. Maintaining the Body's Water Balance

The human body is always working to maintain a delicate balance of water to keep everything running smoothly. The distribution of water occurs in various compartments, encompassing both intracellular spaces within cells and extracellular spaces outside of cells. Understanding the delicate equilibrium of water intake and water loss is crucial for maintaining cellular integrity, balancing electrolyte levels, and supporting overall bodily functions.

3. Indications of Dehydration

Dehydration can be a result of the body losing more fluids than it needs, which can disrupt the delicate balance necessary for optimal functioning. It is crucial to be able to identify the symptoms of dehydration in order to take immediate action. Typical signs and symptoms may include:

Quenching your thirst: Hydration is essential for the body to function properly. Recognizing thirst is an initial sign that the body's hydration is diminishing.

Abnormal Urine Color: Dark yellow urine can be a sign of concentrated waste products resulting from a decrease in water content. Well-hydrated individuals usually have urine that is light yellow or pale in color.

Dehydrated Skin and Mouth: Proper hydration is essential for maintaining healthy skin and preventing dryness in the mouth. Insufficient saliva production can lead to dryness and discomfort.

Feeling tired and lacking energy: Proper hydration is crucial for maintaining optimal blood volume, which ensures that cells receive an adequate supply of oxygen. Without enough fluids, you may experience feelings of fatigue and lethargy.

Headache: Headaches can be caused by dehydration, which reduces blood flow and oxygen supply to the brain.

Feeling lightheaded or dizzy: Insufficient hydration can result in a decrease in blood pressure, leading to feelings of dizziness or lightheadedness.

Reduced Urination: When urine output decreases, it could be a sign of dehydration. This happens because the body tries to save water by producing less urine.

Increased Heart Rate: When the body becomes dehydrated, it may try to compensate for the decrease in blood volume by increasing the heart rate.

4. Factors Affecting Hydration Requirements

It is crucial to consider various factors that can influence individual hydration needs in order to customize fluid intake to specific requirements. Important factors to consider are:

 Age: Hydration needs can vary depending on age, with infants, children, and older adults having different requirements. It is interesting to note that the percentage of body water tends to be higher in children, whereas older adults may sometimes have a diminished sense of thirst.

 Exercise: Strenuous physical activity can cause increased fluid loss, so it's important to drink more water to avoid dehydration. It is crucial for athletes, especially, to be mindful of their hydration levels in order to maximize their performance.

Climate and Temperature: During hot and humid weather, it's important to stay hydrated by drinking more fluids. On the other hand, chilly temperatures can sometimes make it easy to forget about staying hydrated, so it's important to make a conscious effort to drink enough fluids.

Health Conditions: It's important to be aware that certain health conditions, like fever, diarrhea, or vomiting, can lead to increased fluid loss and a higher risk of dehydration. It is important for individuals with kidney or heart conditions to be mindful of their fluid intake.

Dietary Preferences: It's important to note that certain beverages like caffeinated or alcoholic drinks can lead to dehydration, whereas consuming water-rich foods like fruits and vegetables can help maintain proper hydration levels.

5. Best Ways to Stay Hydrated

For individuals looking to stay properly hydrated, there are some practical strategies that can be tailored to their lifestyle and unique requirements. Here are some strategies:

 Importance of Staying Hydrated: It is important to stay hydrated by drinking water regularly, even if you don't feel thirsty. This helps to keep your body's fluid balance in check. Remembering to drink enough water throughout the day is important for maintaining hydration.

 Keeping an Eye on Urine Color: It's important to keep an eye on the color of your urine as it can indicate your hydration levels. When it comes to urine color, a light yellow or pale shade usually means you're well-hydrated. On the other hand, if your urine is dark yellow, it might be a sign that you need to drink more fluids.

Maintaining Electrolyte Balance: When engaging in extended physical activity or experiencing heavy perspiration, particularly in warm environments, it may be important to restore electrolyte levels. One way to achieve this is by consuming sports drinks or foods that are rich in electrolytes.

Including Foods with High Water Content: Including fruits and vegetables with high water content, like watermelon, cucumbers, and oranges, can help keep you hydrated. Adding these foods to your meals and snacks can help you stay hydrated.

Moderating Caffeine and Alcohol Consumption: When it comes to caffeinated and alcoholic beverages, it's important to keep moderation in mind. Consuming them in excess can lead to dehydration. It is advisable to balance the consumption of these beverages with water.

Customizing Hydration for Different Levels of Physical Activity: It is essential to carefully manage your fluid intake in accordance with the intensity and duration of your physical activity. Developing personalized hydration plans can greatly enhance an athlete's performance.

Paying Attention to Your Thirst Signals: Listening to the body's cues for thirst is a natural and effective method for staying hydrated. Drinking water when feeling thirsty is essential for maintaining proper hydration levels in the body.

6. Special Considerations for Populations with Unique Needs

It is important to pay special attention to hydration for the well-being of certain populations who may be more susceptible to dehydration. Some of the groups that are particularly vulnerable include:

For infants and children: Infants and children have a higher surface area to body weight ratio, making them more susceptible to fluid loss. It is important for caregivers to prioritize regular fluid intake, particularly in hot weather or during illnesses.

For Pregnant and Breastfeeding Women: Pregnant and breastfeeding women require increased fluid intake to ensure proper hydration for both themselves and their babies. Proper hydration is crucial for the well-being of both the mother and the baby.

Experienced Individuals: As we get older, our ability to perceive

Dehydration can cause a decrease in thirst and hinder the body's ability to retain water. It is important for older adults to be mindful of their fluid intake in order to avoid dehydration.

People with Chronic Illnesses: Fluid balance can be affected by certain medical conditions, like diabetes or kidney disease. It is important for individuals with chronic illnesses to collaborate with healthcare providers in order to develop suitable hydration plans.

7. Conclusion: The Key to Optimal Well-being

Ultimately, staying properly hydrated is essential for maintaining the delicate balance of physiological functions in the human body. It plays a vital role in overall health, impacting various aspects such as cognitive function and digestive health. Having a good grasp on the signs of dehydration, being able to identify one's unique hydration requirements, and implementing effective strategies for maintaining proper fluid intake can greatly enhance one's ability to prioritize their well-being through conscious hydration.

71

From staying hydrated during a workout to indulging in water-rich fruits for a refreshing snack, making choices that prioritize hydration can greatly enhance one's overall well-being and vitality. Water plays a crucial role in maintaining the optimal functioning of the body's various systems, ensuring overall vitality and well-being. As we recognize the importance of staying hydrated, we acknowledge a crucial aspect of taking care of ourselves—one that resonates throughout our entire being, promoting good health and well-being.

CHAPTER 7

RICE DIET MEAL PLAN

Mastering the art of meal planning can revolutionize your daily dining decisions, leading to improved health, better budgeting, and a significant reduction in food waste. It requires careful planning, meticulous organization, and a deep understanding of nutritional requirements. Discover the numerous advantages of meal planning, learn how to create a well-organized meal plan, master the art of efficient execution, and adapt your meal planning to suit different dietary preferences in this extensive guide.

1. The Advantages of Meal Planning

1.1 Health and Nutrition

Meal planning has a significant impact on improving health and nutrition. Through careful selection of a wide range of nourishing foods, those with expertise in the culinary realm can guarantee that their diet fulfills all necessary vitamin, mineral, and macronutrient needs. Adopting a proactive approach to nutrition can have a positive impact on your overall well-being, assist in maintaining a healthy weight, and potentially lower the risk of chronic diseases.

1.2 Maximizing Efficiency with Your Time

Meal planning is a smart approach that can save you time and make your week more efficient. By strategically planning meals ahead of time, you can save valuable minutes during hectic weekdays. Being knowledgeable about cooking and having all the necessary ingredients on hand can help you avoid making last-minute trips to the grocery store or relying on less nutritious takeout meals.

1.3 Affordable Options

Financial factors frequently influence choices related to food. Planning meals in advance enables individuals to curate a shopping list that aligns with their intended dishes, enabling them to make economical decisions and minimize unnecessary food disposal. Optimizing your grocery shopping and making the most of your ingredients can be a great way to save money while still enjoying delicious meals.

1.4 Minimizing Food Waste

Amidst growing concerns about the environmental consequences of food waste, meal planning has emerged as a sustainable practice. When individuals purchase only the necessary ingredients for their planned meals, they can effectively minimize the spoilage of perishable items and make a positive impact in reducing food waste. This not only has positive impacts on the environment, but also reflects a commitment to responsible and mindful consumption.

2. Simple Steps to Create a Meal Plan

2.1 Evaluating Dietary Goals and Preferences

Prior to delving into meal planning, it is crucial to evaluate one's dietary objectives and personal preferences. Take into account any dietary restrictions, preferences, or specific health objectives. Having a good grasp of these factors will help you make informed decisions about your food choices, whether you're looking to shed some pounds, build muscle, or follow a specific dietary preference like vegetarianism, veganism, or low-carb.

2.2 Choosing Recipes and Creating Diversity

After determining your dietary goals, the next crucial step is choosing the right recipes. It is important to incorporate a wide range of meals into your diet in order to obtain a diverse array of nutrients. It is important to incorporate a variety of nutritious foods into your diet, such as lean proteins, whole grains, fruits, vegetables, and healthy fats. Not only does this enhance nutritional balance, but it also brings a delightful twist to your meals.

2.3 Crafting a Weekly Calendar

Using your expertise in culinary arts, devise a weekly schedule that details the specific dishes to be cooked on each day. Take into account various factors like work schedules, social commitments, and activities that can impact the time you have for meal preparation. An organized schedule is essential for planning meals that are both efficient for busy days and indulgent for relaxed evenings.

2.4 Creating a Shopping List

Using the weekly calendar, create a thorough shopping list. Categorize the list to make your shopping experience more efficient. Group items into categories such as produce, dairy, and proteins. Creating a well-organized list helps to minimize impulsive buying and guarantees that you have all the essential ingredients readily available.

2.5 Mastering the Art of Batch Cooking and Ingredient Prepping

Being efficient is crucial when it comes to planning meals. It's a great idea to prepare larger quantities of certain ingredients that can be utilized in various dishes. For example, you can roast a bunch of vegetables, grill some chicken, or cook a big batch of grains. This streamlines your daily cooking routine and offers ready-to-use components for effortlessly putting together your meals.

Consider the leftovers

Appreciate the potential of leftovers as a crucial element in your meal planning. Prepare generous portions with the foresight of enjoying the leftovers for a delightful meal the following day. This not only saves time but also guarantees that no prepared food is wasted.

3. Strategies for Smooth Implementation

Embrace the power of flexibility.

Having a well-thought-out meal plan is important, but it's also crucial to be open to making adjustments. Life is full of surprises, and unforeseen circumstances or alterations to our plans can happen. It's important to be flexible and willing to make changes to the meal plan if necessary.

3.2 Convenience Planning

Make sure to include convenient options in your meal plan. Opt for convenient and effortless recipes on hectic days, while saving more elaborate meals for moments when there's ample time to prepare. Make the most of your kitchen appliances, such as slow cookers or Instant Pots, to simplify your cooking routines.

3.3 Rotate and Repeat

Meal planning can be made easier by avoiding the need to come up with new ideas every week. Discover cherished recipes and seamlessly integrate them into your culinary repertoire. This streamlines the planning process and guarantees that delightful and well-known meals are included in the weekly rotation.

Utilize technology to your advantage.

Utilize technology to streamline meal planning. There is a wide range of apps and websites available that provide recipe suggestions, help with organizing grocery lists, and even allow you to adjust recipes based on the desired number of servings. These tools are incredibly helpful in streamlining the planning and execution process.

3.5 Make Purposeful Purchases

When grocery shopping, it's important to adhere to your prepared list and resist the temptation of impulsive purchases. Being mindful while shopping not only helps you save money, but also increases the chances of buying items that support your dietary goals.

4. Adjusting Meal Planning to Suit Personal Dietary Preferences
4.1 Meal Planning for Vegetarian and Vegan Diets

When it comes to planning meals for those who follow a vegetarian or vegan lifestyle, it's important to choose a diverse range of plant-based proteins. Think along the lines of beans, lentils, tofu, and tempeh. Indulge in a wide variety of vegetables, fruits, whole grains, and nuts to savor a diverse and nourishing diet.

4.2 Meal Planning for a Low-Carb Diet

For those looking to follow a low-carb diet, it's important to prioritize protein-rich foods like meat, poultry, fish, and eggs. Include a variety of non-starchy vegetables, opt for healthy fats, and enjoy moderate portions of low-carb fruits. Discover a wide range of recipes that cleverly swap out high-carb ingredients for healthier, lower-carb alternatives.

4.3 Meal Planning for a Gluten-Free Diet

When it comes to meal planning, it's important to steer clear of wheat, barley, and rye if you're looking for a gluten-free diet. Discover the wonders of naturally gluten-free grains such as quinoa, rice, and oats (if certified gluten-free). Experiment with gluten-free flours for baking and discover a variety of vegetables, proteins, and dairy options that are naturally free of gluten.

4.4 Meal Planning for the Mediterranean Diet

Following a Mediterranean diet means including lean proteins, whole grains, olive oil, and plenty of fruits and vegetables. Consider incorporating fish, nuts, and legumes into your diet to boost your protein intake. It is important to focus on incorporating fresh and minimally processed foods into your diet, while also reducing your consumption of red meat and processed items.

5. Conclusion: Changing Your Eating Habits for a Lifetime

Ultimately, becoming skilled in the craft of meal planning can lead to a significant shift in developing wholesome and eco-friendly dietary practices. Meal planning goes beyond just saving time and money. It sets the stage for a well-rounded and purposeful approach to eating. It enables people to make informed decisions about their food, in line with their health objectives and dietary preferences.

With meal planning becoming a regular practice, it goes beyond being just a daily task and transforms into a way of life that embraces the pleasure of cooking, the skill of nourishing the body, and the fulfillment of minimizing food waste. Through the careful curation of each meal, people embark on a journey of self-nurturing, fostering a deep connection with the nourishment that not only fuels their bodies but also uplifts their spirits. Meal planning takes on a crucial role in the symphony of daily life, ensuring a harmonious blend of health, well-being, and culinary delight.

THE END